Demystifying PTSD

A Guide Book for PTSD Victims
and Their Loved Ones

By

Dr. David A. Jones

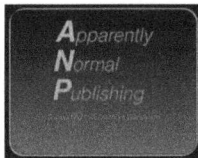

Apparently
Normal
Publishing

Apparently Normal Publishing

Demystifying PTSD

Cover designed by Dr. David A. Jones.
Cover art and photography:
Used under license from iStockphoto.com or Shutterstock.com.

Published by:
Apparently Normal Publishing
Waterloo, Ontario, Canada

ISBN (Paperback Edition): 978-0-9951963-0-8
Version 2016/07/28

Acknowledgments

Demystifying PTSD is the result of a journey that started for me while I was in Graduate School at the University of Western Ontario. I'd like to express my thanks to my graduate supervisor, Gary Rollman, for all of his wisdom and patience, and for encouraging me to think outside the prevailing Cognitive Behavioural box. I am also grateful for the guidance I received from two very gifted psychologists and teachers, Jack Sweetland and Elizabeth Werth, who opened my eyes to the richness of Object Relations Theory and psychodynamic concepts. Most of all, I owe an enormous debt of gratitude to Roger Solomon and Kathy Martin, who enriched my EMDR skills by opening up the world of Structural Dissociation Theory in their Art of EMDR workshops.

Waterloo, Ontario

June, 2016

Other Books by Dr. David A. Jones

Fiction
(Writing as Alex Jones)

WALLS: The Identity Trilogy, Book One

FACES: The Identity Trilogy, Book Two

ANGELA'S EYES: The Identity Trilogy, Prequel

Find out more about the Alex Jones Identity Trilogy at:
http://alex-jones-author.com

Table of Contents

List of Tables

List of Figures

Introduction

In the first five years after I graduated with my Ph.D. from the University of Western Ontario (now known as Western University) and started practicing psychology, I became aware of three very important trends in my practice. First, I realized that a large number of clients who came to me with previous diagnoses of severe anxiety and depression, were actually suffering from Posttraumatic Stress Disorder (PTSD). Second, the Cognitive Behavioral Therapy (CBT) skills that I learned in graduate school were not working nearly as well as I would have liked for these clients. Third, the way these PTSD victims presented in real life was very different than the picture of PTSD that was painted by DSM-IV, the prevailing diagnostic standard in North America at that time.

One of the most common things I noticed in PTSD victims was how upset these people were with themselves for not being able to "just get over it". Most of them had been functioning well in their jobs and their relationships before they experienced the trauma that triggered their PTSD. But suddenly, everything had fallen apart for them. They were baffled as to why they were completely unable to cope with stress anymore, and why they couldn't put their trauma behind them. I noticed that most of these victims beat themselves up badly because they felt weak and defective, when they had previously felt strong and confident. As a result, these people became even more anxious and depressed over their inability to solve the mystery of what had happened to them.

Even worse, the relationships of most of these PTSD victims with their family and friends had deteriorated badly. I noticed that victims had little tolerance for any kind of sensory or emotional stimulation. They became incredibly irritable and tended to push their loved ones away. Their families and loved ones were mystified about what had happened to the person they knew before the trauma, and they were losing patience with them. PTSD was destroying the lives of these PTSD victims and it was tearing their marriages, relationships, and friendships apart.

At that point in time, I started looking for new psychological tools to improve my ability to help these unfortunate trauma victims. A few years before this, I had heard about a new therapy known as Eye Movement Desensitization and Reprocessing (EMDR). My initial reaction at the time was that EMDR sounded like the psychology equivalent of snake oil in a travelling medicine show. But my curiosity got the better of me as time went on, and I did some research on EMDR. I found a surprising number of reports that supported the new therapy as being an effective treatment for PTSD, so I figured that I might as well find out for myself what it was all about. I registered for the Level One EMDR Training in Vancouver in November 2005, and I began trying out the new therapy when I returned home.

Almost immediately, EMDR therapy opened my eyes to the real world of PTSD. I began to see the dynamic

mental processes of my clients unfold before my eyes, and I began to see PTSD in a very different way. Buoyed by my new enthusiasm, I took the Level Two EMDR Training in Calgary six months later.

Fast forward five years, and I now had five years of experience using EMDR to treat PTSD. About this time, I stumbled upon an online article by Dr. J. Douglas Bremner[25], a psychiatrist and researcher, who described PTSD as being a disease that disrupts the normal processing of memories in our brain. The article immediately struck a chord with me, because that's what my EMDR training had taught me, and it's exactly what I had seen repeatedly in the PTSD victims I had treated over the previous five years. As I thought about Dr. Bremner's article, I began to see similarities between how my PTSD clients described their impaired cognitive functioning, and how my computer acted when its performance slowed down drastically. As I thought about it more, a model of PTSD started forming in my mind, using computers as the analogy for what I saw happening in the brains of the people I treated with PTSD.

Shortly afterwards, I began using that analogy of PTSD to explain the disorder to clients. I was surprised to see how quickly my clients latched onto the model. I began hearing the same thing over and over from them: "That's exactly how I feel. I wish you could explain that to my (husband, wife, or family)." These people had entered my office feeling overwhelmed, hopeless, and abandoned by the mental health system, and often also by their loved ones. But now they were leaving the office with a new sense of hope. Now that they had an explanation for how their brain had become overwhelmed, they were able to begin the process of not blaming themselves for their disorder. They now had hope that their PTSD could be reversed with appropriate psychological treatments such as EMDR.

Since then, I have used my information processing analogy to explain PTSD to hundreds of new clients. In situations where marital or family strife at home threatens my client's stability, I often invite loved ones to a session where I use the model to explain PTSD to them. More often than not, these people leave my office with a new understanding of PTSD and a new appreciation for how their loved one has been affected by the disorder. It helps loved ones to be more tolerant and supportive of their family members while the victims move through their therapy. Since social supports tend to reduce the stress in the PTSD victim's lives, educating families makes my job – treating their loved one's PTSD – that much easier.

Because the *Information Processing Model* has been so helpful for my PTSD clients and their families, I've written this book to share it with you – people who either have PTSD yourself, or have a loved one who is struggling with the disorder. Even though PTSD is a highly complex disorder, I've tried to describe it as simply as possible. I've purposely avoided burdening you with too many scientific terms or too much scientific research. Where I have included references, it is to give credit to important researchers in the history of psychology, or to direct you to some additional resources. Many of the references are from

Wikipedia, since that site gives you a quick overview of many of the concepts in this book. However, if you're hungry for more information on that subject, simply follow the links from Wikipedia, or use your web browser to explore the topics in as much depth as you prefer.

Hopefully this book will give you the information you need to help you and your loved ones better understand PTSD. With information and understanding comes hope for improvement in the future. Thus, the final chapter of this book is devoted to helping you find the most appropriate types of mental health programs and professionals for treating your unique PTSD symptoms. It may still be a challenge for many of you to find adequate treatment. However, it is my hope that the information in this book will give you the hope and patience to rise to that challenge, and help you to reclaim the future that you envisioned for yourselves and your families.

Chapter One: The Need for Education

Posttraumatic Stress Disorder, or PTSD as it is commonly known, is one of the least understood and mysterious of all mental health disorders. Most of us may hear about it on the evening news, usually in relation to soldiers or first responders who witness horrific, traumatizing events. But what most people don't know, is that PTSD is all around us and is much more common than we think. It afflicts people who have been traumatized by a wide range of common events like domestic abuse and violence, workplace harassment, workplace accidents, or automobile accidents, to name a few.

PTSD is a disorder where previously well-functioning individuals, many of whom formerly thought of themselves as being emotionally strong and tough, suffer a complete emotional breakdown after experiencing one or more traumatic events. They find themselves overcome with anxiety and depression. Suddenly, they become completely unable to function or cope with daily life.

Victims of PTSD cannot figure out what has happened to them. They become angry, despondent, withdrawn and depressed over their inability to pull their lives back together. But even worse, the very people that PTSD victims rely on for empathy and support – their families and loved ones – are just as bewildered and frustrated by the person's sudden inability to cope with life. Victims begin to feel like their families don't understand them and are abandoning them. Both the victims and their families become desperate to find somebody who can help the affected person.

When PTSD sufferers reach out for help, they are often initially diagnosed with some kind of anxiety disorder, depressive disorder, or both. They will usually receive whatever limited counselling their health plans or community services provide for people with anxiety and depression, usually with little improvement. PTSD victims know they need something more, but they don't know where to go. They soon become desperate to find somebody who understands their situation and can help them.

Ultimately, many PTSD victims become disillusioned, becoming increasingly withdrawn, antisocial, and hopeless about their future. The rate of suicide in PTSD victims is high, as evidenced by frequent news reports about veterans who return home and take their own lives when they don't receive the help they need.

During the course of my job as a psychologist, one of the biggest challenges I face with clients who seek treatment for PTSD, is to give them hope that they can become well again. Giving them hope is essential, since before people can begin the long journey to overcome PTSD, they must first understand the nature of the beast that they are fighting. And equally as important, their spouses and families must also understand what their loved one is going through in order to provide emotional support while victims go through their treatment journey.

Soon after I began taking extra professional training

for treating PTSD, I recognized the enormous need for education to help PTSD victims and their families understand PTSD. So, over the years, I've brought together the things I've learned in my training and combined them with my clinical observations of hundreds of PTSD victims, to create a model that helps people to finally understand what has happened to them as a result of the traumatic events they have experienced. The model I've developed resonates with my clients. The look on their faces when they realize that somebody has finally understood and validated what they are going through, is priceless – it is the first ray of hope they have had since they suffered their emotional breakdown.

The model I share with my clients, which I am going to share with you in this book, is not based on neuroscience or technical psycho-babble. It is based on clinical observation. It brings PTSD down to earth, explaining it in a way that resonates with ordinary, everyday people everywhere, making it easy to understand.

Chapter Two: Your Brain Before PTSD

UNDERSTANDING NORMAL INFORMATION PROCESSING

Personal Computing Devices	Tasks	Our Brains
Keyboard, Mouse, Touchscreen, Microphone, CD or DVD, Camera, Internet	Information Input	Our senses (hearing, sight, touch, taste, smell), internal organs, and emotions
RAM	Temporary Storage	Short Term Memory
CPU and specialized chips (Video processing, etc)	Information Processing	Cerebral Cortex and Subcortex
Hard Drives, USB Drives, Writeable CD or DVD, Internet 'Cloud' Servers	Output & Long Term Storage	Long Term Memory

Table 1: Information Processing

Before we can use any model to understand how PTSD works, our model needs to first explain how our brain works normally when we don't have PTSD. And perhaps the best way to understand how our brain functions, is to compare it to something we use every day – the computers, smart phones, and tablets that have become an essential part of our lives. These different forms of personal computing devices all perform the same important tasks as our brains, as you can see from Table 1.

INFORMATION INPUT

Like our brains, phones, tablets, and computers all take in information from the world around us. Our computing devices do this in the same way that our brains take in information from all of our senses – what we see, hear, feel, taste, smell, and what we feel emotionally. But instead of having senses, our devices receive information that we input from a keyboard, mouse, touchscreen, microphone, CD or DVD, or from the Internet.

TEMPORARY STORAGE

After the information is inside our devices, they need to process or change that information in some way that is useful in our daily lives. To do so, we open a computer program or an "app" on our smartphone or tablet, so that we can write our essay, calculate our budget or taxes, or edit our pictures or videos so we can post them in messages to our friends. And in order for the apps to do so, our devices need to have a temporary storage area to hold the information while our devices process or alter it in some way. In our personal devices, we call this area *Random Access Memory*, or *RAM* for short. In our brains, we simply call it *Short Term Memory*. As we will see in a moment, this temporary storage area is the most important part of both our brain and our personal computing devices.

INFORMATION PROCESSING

Processing information is what our brains and our personal computing devices are all about. This is where our brains and our devices interpret the information that is coming in, and then use that information to perform an important task. In our brains, that task may be trying to understand what we're seeing or what somebody is saying to us, or it may be trying to solve a problem at school or at work. Our brain may be scanning our nerve endings to see if the object that we're touching is too hot or too cold to touch or to eat. In order to process the information as we hold it in our Short Term Memory, we use many areas of our brain's cerebral cortex and subcortex to understand and interpret the incoming information. In our computing devices, the task of understanding, interpreting, and using the incoming information is performed by a computer chip known as the *Central Processing Unit*, or *CPU* for short. The CPU is the brain of our personal devices. Although our phone, tablet, or computer may also have other specialized chips for processing information like graphics (photographs and video), all of this information ultimately ends up being analyzed by the device's brain – the CPU.

OUTPUT AND LONG TERM STORAGE

The end goal of information processing, both in our brains and in our personal computing devices, is to take the result of information processing, and to send the information somewhere to store it, so we can recall it or share the information later with other people. In our brains, once the incoming information is understood or processed, it is sent to *Long Term Memory* areas of the brain so that we can remember and use that information in the future. In humans, we think this normal process of moving and storing information in Long Term Memory may occur at night when we're sleeping, especially during our periods of deepest sleep, which we call *Rapid Eye Movement* or *REM* sleep. In our personal computing devices, the information is moved to permanent storage devices such as hard drives, USB flash drives, writeable CD's or DVD's, or to large computer servers on the Internet called *Cloud Servers*.

THE IMPORTANCE OF SHORT TERM MEMORY & RAM

If we use computers, tablets, or smart phones at all, we all know what happens when we ask our device to do too much – when we have too many apps running at once, or if we try to make a video or movie that is too long or complex for the device. All of a sudden, we notice that our device starts getting slower and slower – we may see the little color wheel on Mac computers, or the hourglass on PC computers, that tells us to wait while our devices try to shuffle information around in its short-term RAM memory, so it can finish processing the information. The smaller the amount of RAM in our device, the more likely the device will start slowing down. Sometimes it may actually "hang" and stop working entirely. While this can be incredibly annoying when we're using our computer or mobile devices, it isn't usually catastrophic and we don't usually lose too much information. All we have to do is turn off the device and "reboot" or turn it back on again in order to clear the short term RAM memory. Then we simply start our task again from scratch.

If we compare our brains to our computing devices, we know that exactly the same thing can happen to our brains. We can all remember times when we've had difficulty concentrating or hearing somebody who is talking to us, when we're also trying to do something else at the same time, or if there is too much other commotion going on around us. The more information that is coming into our brains at one time, the more inefficient our brain becomes. It becomes unable to keep up with the new information, and unable to understand and process it. And if the amount of information coming into our brain through all of our senses and emotions is completely overwhelming, our brains can slow down, become completely overwhelmed, and "hang" just like our personal computing devices.

INFORMATION OVERLOAD AND PTSD

The big problem with the human brain is that we can't just reboot or restart our brain, like we can with our personal computing devices. When our brain becomes overwhelmed by information overload, our ability to process information can break down completely. This is exactly what we see happening to people who experience one or more severe emotional traumas – a situation that we now call Posttraumatic Stress Disorder (PTSD). In other words, PTSD is a state where we see a person's normal capacity for information processing become completely overwhelmed, so that the person's brain has a greatly reduced ability to process any new information or emotional stimulation.

Chapter Three: Diagnosing PTSD

You or your loved ones may already suspect that you might have PTSD, but you may be asking yourselves: *How do I find out if I have PTSD or not?* The short answer is that it may be more difficult than you think to find somebody who can properly answer this question and give you a proper diagnosis. In reality, however, the reasons for why it is so difficult to confirm or rule out whether you have PTSD, are more complex.

One major reason for the difficulty in diagnosing PTSD is that the public was largely unaware of the existence of the disorder until recently. Unless you had experienced a severe life trauma and were diagnosed with PTSD, or unless you were a family member or loved one of somebody affected by PTSD, you were probably unaware of its existence. In recent years, however, news reports about PTSD in the media have been increasing in number and public awareness is slowly on the rise.

Recently, people have seen more frequent news reports about the high incidence of PTSD in soldiers returning from wars in Iraq, Afghanistan, or Vietnam, or about the millions of refugees who are fleeing civil war in the Middle East. We're also starting to hear more reports of the toll that PTSD is taking on our first responders: police, firefighters, and paramedics. But despite the increase in reports about PTSD, there are still a large number of incorrect myths about the disorder that often result in the disorder going undiagnosed. For example, it's often assumed that PTSD only occurs after a single, devastating traumatic experience such as a gruesome battle, a major natural disaster, or from being raped or beaten. Even worse, there are many who don't believe that PTSD even exists. Those people believe that victims of the disorder just need to "suck it up and move on."

So, if there is still such a lack of understanding about PTSD, how does one know if we have the disorder or not? How does a psychiatrist or psychologist actually go about diagnosing a person with PTSD? Why does it often go undiagnosed? One way of answering these questions is found in standardized sets of diagnostic criteria that have been developed by bodies such as the American Psychiatric Association (APA) and the World Health Organization (WHO). In North America, psychiatrists and psychologists generally tend to use the APA diagnostic manual, which is called DSM-5,[1] while the rest of the world tends to use the WHO diagnostic criteria known as ICD-10.[2]

DSM-5 DIAGNOSTIC CRITERIA

The DSM-5 criteria for diagnosing PTSD consist of five major groups of symptoms, plus three additional separate criteria, which must all be met in order for a person to be diagnosed with PTSD. If we break down the diagnostic groups, we can see a pattern emerge that allows us to lump the symptoms together into four distinct clusters that explain and define PTSD. The first cluster is a group of symptoms that is very similar to those seen in major depressive disorders. The second cluster is a group of symptoms of fear, anxiety, and avoidance that is usually seen in various Anxiety Disorders. The third cluster is a group of symptoms that describes the state of sensory and emotional overload that is the important trademark of PTSD, which I described in Chapter Two. Finally, the fourth symptom cluster is known as Dissociative Symptoms. This cluster of symptoms arises either from the brain's attempt to avoid remembering traumatic memories, or from the brain's inability to forget those traumatic events.

ICD-10 DIAGNOSTIC CRITERIA

The WHO diagnostic criteria in ICD-10 are not as extensive as those in DSM-5. But in some respects, ICD-10 better reflects the Information Processing model of PTSD that I proposed in Chapter Two (Your Brain Before PTSD). ICD-10 contains one large group of symptoms that defines the sensory and emotional overload and hyper-arousal that I described in our model. Like DSM-5, ICD-10 also acknowledges the fear, anxiety, and avoidance that exist in PTSD. And also like DSM-5, the ICD-10 criteria include references to the dissociative symptoms that occur when the brain reaches a state of overload. Although ICD-10 mentions that anxiety and depression are common when people have PTSD, there is much less emphasis on anxiety and depressive symptoms, and much more emphasis on the hyper-arousal and dissociative symptoms of PTSD.

PROBLEMS WITH DIAGNOSTIC CRITERIA

Although standardized Diagnostic Criteria are essential for providing standards for diagnosing PTSD, they also create some significant problems. One of the major difficulties in diagnosing PTSD in North America is the over-reliance on DSM-5 criteria for diagnosing the disorder, in combination with a dire shortage of skilled therapists who are specially trained for recognizing the hyper-arousal and dissociative symptoms of the disorder.

The vast majority of psychiatrists, psychologists, social workers, and behavior therapists are well trained in recognizing the symptoms of various anxiety and depressive disorders that are the most common mental health problems. So when those professionals do their initial evaluations of people who might be suffering from PTSD, they only tend to look for the symptoms they see most often on a daily basis – anxiety and depression. Unfortunately, while anxiety and depression may be the most commonly seen symptoms of PTSD, they are often caused by more serious symptoms that are easily overlooked unless we are trained to look for them – the hyper-arousal and dissociative clusters of symptoms.

A good analogy for this phenomenon is the iceberg shown in Figure 1. As survivors of the Titanic disaster learned, it's not the small, beautiful part of the iceberg above the water that causes problems. It's the majority of the iceberg lurking beneath the water that is so deadly. Symptoms of anxiety and depression are like the visible tip of the iceberg, while hyper-arousal and dissociation make up the bulk of the PTSD iceberg beneath the surface that so often goes unseen.

As a result, vast numbers of people who have been badly traumatized are diagnosed with various anxiety or depressive disorders, when they should really be diagnosed with PTSD. And even more tragically, their treatment then focuses only on the tip of the PTSD iceberg - anxiety and depression - but fails to address the underlying hyper-arousal and dissociation that prolong their misery unless they are properly treated.

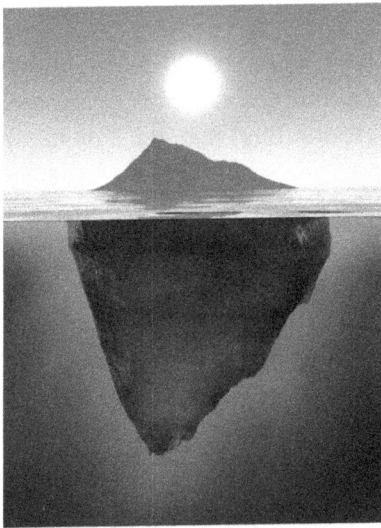

Figure 1: Dissociation Compared to an Iceberg

Another major problem with using diagnostic criteria, especially DSM-5, is that people often think that *all* of the criteria apply to *everybody* who has been diagnosed with PTSD. In short, they often think that everybody with PTSD is affected in the same way. But in reality, exactly the opposite is true. Because there are an endless number of ways in which people can be traumatized, and because everybody reacts differently to those terrifying events, *PTSD is unique and different for every single person who is affected by the disorder.* So, unfortunately, the unique nature and severity of PTSD in individuals is not captured in either DSM-5 or ICD-10 diagnostic criteria, and the diagnosis is often missed.

OUR INFORMATION PROCESSING MODEL

In contrast to Diagnostic Criteria like DSM-5 and ICD-10, the Information Processing model of PTSD that I presented in Chapter Two, better describes the nature and intensity of PTSD for each person. The model does that by focusing primarily on the extent of information overload and associated hyper-arousal, and on the severity and unique characteristics of each person's dissociative symptoms. Clinicians who are specially trained to diagnose and treat PTSD truly understand the importance of information overload, hyper-arousal, and dissociation. They tend to focus more on those symptoms when investigating whether or not a person might have PTSD, rather than relying exclusively on diagnostic criteria such as DSM-5 or ICD-10.

Our model of PTSD, *defined as a state where people's capacity to process information has been overloaded by one or many traumatic events*, helps people understand why they are unable to keep their brain focused on what is happening in the moment, and why they get stuck reliving and remembering their traumas over and over again. The model also helps people understand why their brains manage to find ways to push things away or to escape from reality, in order to prevent any further information overload and to prevent becoming stuck in reliving their traumatic past.

Because the process of dissociation is such a huge part of the PTSD iceberg, and because it plays such an important role in PTSD, it deserves a separate discussion in Chapter Four, where we will try to help people understand what is happening when they dissociate, and why they dissociate in the first place. If we're going to be successful in treating PTSD and eliminating the state of information overload, we must first treat the dissociative symptoms of the disorder. The beauty of this approach is that if we're successful, the anxiety and depressive symptoms that make up the tip of the PTSD iceberg will eventually melt away on their own once we properly treat the dissociative symptoms below the water and they disappear.

Chapter Four: What is Dissociation?

The biggest problem in explaining dissociation is that, even though psychiatrists and some psychologists have talked about it for over a century, there has been very little systematic research on dissociation since the early 1900's. To fully understand why that happened, I would have to give you a long lesson in the history of both psychiatry and psychology over the past century. To make a long story short, suffice it to say that psychological research went in a totally different direction during the 20th century, with the evolution of Behaviorism[3] and Cognitive Psychology. [4]

However, beginning in the 1990's, psychologist's interest in emotions and dissociation was rekindled, particularly with advances such as Les Greenburg's *Emotion Focused Therapy* and Francine Shapiro's *Eye Movement Desensitization and Reprocessing (EMDR) Therapy*. This was especially true of mental health practitioners who were treating people with histories of severe trauma and abuse, since they were looking for more effective ways to treat people with traumatic histories. With this new focus on emotions, modern researchers such as Onno van der Hart and his colleagues revived interest in Pierre Janet's work on dissociation from the early 1900's.[5] In their book, *The Haunted Self,*[6] van der Hart and colleagues talk about how difficult it is to accurately define dissociation, precisely because there has been so little research on the subject, and because everyone in the trauma field uses the term differently.

If that's the case, let's at least try to paint a simple picture of dissociation that most of us can understand. Back in the early 1900's, Janet initially described dissociation as multiple unconscious mental processes, split off from each other, that can function separately at the same time. When I say that, I know the first thing that pops into your head – the words *Multiple Personalities* and the 1976 TV mini-series *Sybil*.[7] Because these labels are commonly used to describe people with a severe mental health problem, we immediately jump to the conclusion that dissociation is a very dangerous phenomenon. But, in fact, multiple personalities are extremely rare and they only occur in the most severe cases of trauma and dissociation.

WHEN IS DISSOCIATION A GOOD THING?

Unlike severe mental health states like multiple personalities, the split mental states described by Janet can sometimes be healthy, normal occurrences in our daily lives. For example, there are times when it is perfectly normal to feel love, anger, fear, caring, and loving. There are also times when it is perfectly natural to run, hide, or fight in the face of danger. To visualize this, take a look at the image in Figure 2.

We can think of each separate mental state as if it was a separate room inside our brain. When we're healthy, we're able to open the doors and move easily from room to room, so that our various mental states work together in a coordinated fashion. When this happens, we are living in a state of mental integration, where we are able to access the most appropriate mental states for any given situation, and we are not overwhelmed by the information in those mental states.

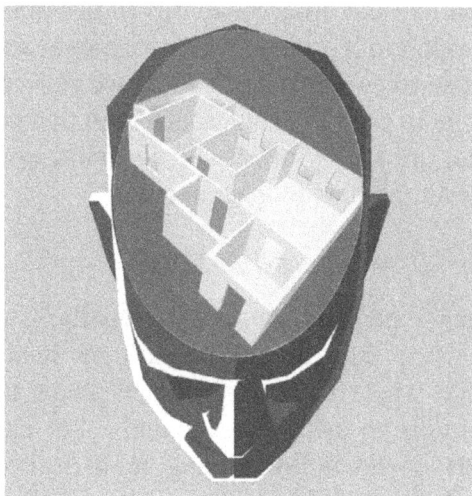

Figure 2: Healthy Dissociation

Let's look at an example that most of us are familiar with. We've all had times when our minds have wandered while we're driving. Suddenly we realize that we've driven for five or ten minutes without having an accident, but we don't even remember how we got to our present location. In this case, our mind has split into an unconscious function that remembers how to drive a car properly, while allowing another part of our mind to think about something else. Similarly, we've all had times when we feel extremely sad over the loss of a loved one or a pet, but we still manage to function, almost like a robot, in most of our daily activities while we continue to grieve. In both cases, we are able to access two rooms in our brain at the same time so that we can multi-task more efficiently. The truth is, when we are healthy, we all have many different roles and emotional states, much like the different rooms in our brain in Figure 2. More importantly, we're able to move automatically between those roles and states, so that we can be the person we need to be in each life situation. When that happens, our mental states are highly integrated and mild dissociation is a perfectly natural, healthy phenomenon.

WHEN IS DISSOCIATION UNHEALTHY?

When people are emotionally traumatized, especially when they are children, they tend to escape mentally into whatever mental process helps to make the painful emotion go away most quickly. For children, that often means daydreaming, hiding in their bedrooms, or trying to please parents or abusers in an effort to avoid more abuse and more painful emotions. Because it tends to help them avoid pain, people start to depend on these styles of coping rigidly and exclusively, which interferes with their ability to cope by using other healthier coping styles or emotional states. In effect, if we think in terms of the image in Figure 2, traumatized people either get stuck, or they lock themselves into, one single room in their brain that represents one traumatic mental state.

Over long periods of time, trauma victims remain stuck in various unhealthy emotional states, such as fear or helplessness, or in unhealthy coping styles such as avoidance or perfectionism, that help them to avoid their painful emotions. The more often a person becomes stuck in one or more of these emotional states, and the less they are able to move freely into healthier roles or emotional states, the more severe their dissociation becomes.

INFORMATION OVERLOAD AND DISSOCIATION

So, now that you know a bit about dissociation, you're probably asking: How does this relate to our model of PTSD and information overload? The answer is that dissociation appears to be our brain's natural response for trying to protect us from situations where it is becoming overloaded with emotional and sensory information. If we think in terms of the mental rooms in our brain in Figure 2, dissociation locks us into one room (mental state) at a time. This helps to simplify our world, thus protecting us from being overloaded by the information that has flooded into the other rooms (other mental states).

DISSOCIATION AS A CONTINUUM

Because we've seen how dissociation can be a perfectly healthy emotional state, but can also be a severe mental health problem, it is helpful to see dissociation on a continuum that ranges from very mild to severe. As you can see from Figure 3, simple phobias (such as the fear of heights, closed spaces or spiders) occur as a result of relatively mild dissociation. In the case of phobias, a person gets stuck frequently in a needless state of fear, and we call it *Primary Dissociation*. However, as a person's dissociation becomes more severe, their PTSD symptoms also become more complex and we call it *Secondary Dissociation*. Finally, when dissociation becomes so severe that a person develops more than one distinct personality, we call it *Tertiary Dissociation.*

Dissociation Severity

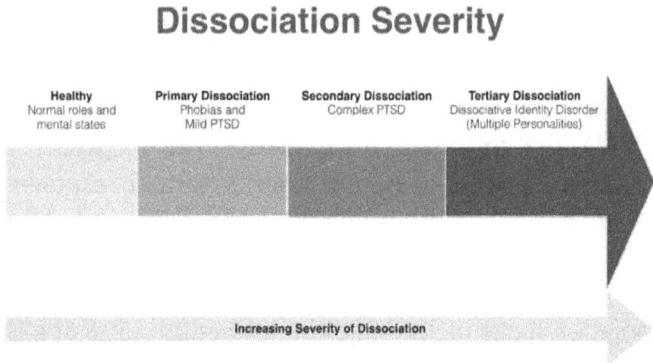

Figure 3: Dissociation Severity

WHY THE DISTINCTION?

At this point, you're probably wondering why the distinction between *Primary, Secondary, and Tertiary Dissociation* is important. The answer is quite simple. The type of treatment you need, and how long your treatment will take, depends entirely on how badly stuck you are in unhealthy, unconscious mental states, and on how severe your dissociative symptoms are. Knowing more about dissociation will help you and your loved ones to better understand how to find the treatment that is most appropriate and helpful for the severity of your unique PTSD symptoms.

Chapter Five: Treatment of PTSD

So far in this book, we've developed a model where we see PTSD as being a state of information overload that causes the brain to dissociate in varying degrees, much like modern computing devices when their memory becomes overwhelmed. We've also learned how this state of information overload negatively affects your short-term memory and your ability to focus and concentrate on new information. More importantly, we've learned that the severity of your PTSD symptoms depends largely on the severity of your dissociative symptoms. In Chapter Four, we saw how dissociation can occur on a continuum from mild to very severe, resulting in PTSD that can also range from being mild to very severe.

So, now that we have a model that gives you a basic understanding of PTSD, we finally get to the most important issue for you: *How can I get some treatment that will finally make me better?*

I would love to be able to give each and every one of you a simple answer that would cover your unique PTSD treatment needs. However, in reality, finding treatment for PTSD can be a "Good News, Bad News" scenario. The good news is that there are a number of different treatments that are all appropriate for treating different degrees of PTSD, and advances and improvements continue to be made in treating PTSD. The bad news is that it can often be difficult to access those treatments. Finding the right treatment for you depends on many different factors, including the severity and chronicity of your unique dissociative symptoms, but also on many other socioeconomic factors.

SYMPTOM MANAGEMENT

Before we discuss treatments for PTSD in detail, we need to make a distinction between learning how to *manage* your PTSD symptoms from day to day, versus longer-term *treatment* that will effectively reduce your dissociative symptoms, and gradually relieve the state of information overload that your brain has been experiencing with PTSD.

Because your mind is in a constant state of overload when you have PTSD, it is vital that you are constantly working to reduce the amount of stimulation and information coming into your brain. You can do this by having a mental health professional teach you some *Stabilization Skills*, including relaxation, meditation, mindfulness, or anchoring skills.

Since being in a state of relaxation, meditation, or mindfulness is the exact opposite of being anxious and over-stimulated, it is physically impossible for you to be both relaxed and anxious at the same time. In terms of our Information Processing Model of PTSD, learning to relax or meditate is the equivalent of shutting down some mental processes that are contributing to your mental overload. This is similar to what we would do if we gradually shut down some unnecessary apps on our computers or smartphones when their processing slows down. Once you are relaxed, it is important to prevent any additional dissociation and overload by learning to focus your mind, and to anchor it back on the present time and present place while you continue to relax.

At some point in your attempts to deal with PTSD, your family physician or a psychiatrist may have prescribed medications for you. People often make the mistake of thinking that those medications are a treatment for PTSD, and that they might eventually help their symptoms to go away. Just as learning relaxation and stabilization skills are important tools for learning to manage your PTSD symptoms, medications are another useful tool that can also help to reduce the severity of your PTSD symptoms. Clinically, medications help to keep you more calm and they help to reduce the state of information overload in your brain. They are another tool in your toolbox of strategies for *managing* your symptoms while you are receiving proven forms of PTSD therapy, or while you are waiting to find appropriate treatment. However, you should not fall into the trap of thinking that your medications are an effective treatment for PTSD – I have yet to see one person with PTSD whose symptoms have disappeared because of the medications they have been taking.

Until you receive appropriate long-term treatment for your PTSD symptoms, you will have to rely on medications or use your stabilization skills frequently, often many times every day, to manage your brain's constant state of information overload. You will also have to use these skills frequently while you are receiving treatment for PTSD, until your symptoms start to subside.

TYPES OF PTSD TREATMENT

Because treatments for PTSD have gradually developed and evolved over the past century, and also because our treatments for PTSD have become more complex over time, I'm going to discuss them in the order in which they were developed. As it turns out, our oldest forms of psychological treatment are usually the least complex, and they are best suited for milder forms of PTSD with less severe dissociation. On the other hand, our newer psychological treatments are more complex and are better suited for more complex forms of PTSD and cases of multiple personalities.

I'm not going to describe all of the available treatments in depth. For those of you who are interested in learning more about their history and development, see the *Appendix* at the back of this book. Understanding more about the history of psychology and psychological treatments will aid your understanding of why certain treatments are better suited to treating PTSD than others.

DESENSITIZATION (EXPOSURE THERAPY)

Systematic Desensitization [8] is one of the oldest, and perhaps the most proven and effective, psychological tool we have. It was developed during the age of Behavioral Psychology, and it is still used extensively today in the treatment of anxiety, phobias, and mild PTSD. Its premise is very simple. We teach people to face their fears (*exposure*) in a gradual manner, while teaching them to relax (*desensitization)* at the same time in the feared situation. By repeating this process over and over, people gradually learn to overcome their fears in a systematic fashion.

Because we are human and we have thoughts (cognitions) about our fears, psychologists have also added elements of Cognitive Therapy, [9] which was developed during the 1950's and 1960's. The addition of cognitive elements has made Systematic Desensitization even more effective. While people learn to relax in situations where they have learned to be afraid, psychologists or psychotherapists also teach them to reprogram their thinking so they can learn that there is really nothing to fear in that situation. This allows the desensitization therapy to proceed more quickly.

The advantages of Systematic Desensitization therapy are that it is a highly effective way of treating phobias and mild PTSD. Most mental health workers, whether they be psychiatrists, psychologists, social workers, or psychotherapists, have been trained to do this type of therapy. The biggest disadvantage of Systematic Desensitization is that it is much less effective, and potentially dangerous, if used too soon with people who are suffering from complex PTSD. In those cases, exposure can potentially overwhelm and re-traumatize people who have high levels of dissociative symptoms, if it is used before the dissociative symptoms are sufficiently reduced. Overall, Systematic Desensitization is best suited for treating phobias and cases of mild PTSD.

COGNITIVE BEHAVIORAL THERAPY (CBT)

Cognitive psychologists believe that our behavior

and our emotions are driven by our thoughts. They believe that by changing how we think about a situation, we can change our emotional response, and we can choose to change how we act in that situation. Because Cognitive Behavioral research dominated psychology from the late 1950's to the 1990's, a great deal of scientific evidence accumulated to show the overall effectiveness of Cognitive Behavioral Therapy [10] in reducing people's psychological distress.

An unfortunate side effect of the dominance of psychology by Cognitive Behavioral psychologists is that people began to believe that CBT was the *only* evidence-based therapy that was effective in treating most mental health disorders. Another incorrect assumption of CBT is that it is effective in treating even the most severe psychological disorders. In situations where CBT hasn't been effective, it has often been assumed that patients or their personalities have somehow been to blame for their lack of treatment progress, instead of questioning the effectiveness of CBT. Over time, however, more and more mental health professionals began to notice the shortcomings of CBT in treating more complex forms of PTSD and other mental health disorders, and they began searching for more effective forms of treatment for PTSD.

The primary advantage of CBT is that it is widely researched and widely available, since most mental health professionals have been trained to use CBT as their primary form of treatment. One disadvantage of CBT is that there has never been one single, standardized form of CBT. There are as many variations of CBT, all based on basic

Cognitive Behavior theory, as there are different CBT therapists. Some therapists adhere strictly to CBT theory, while other more eclectic therapists may use some CBT principles for treating some patients, while mixing it with other forms of therapy for treating other people.

Another major disadvantage of CBT is that many agencies have devised "cookie cutter" CBT treatment programs that are designed to provide the same treatment to everybody who comes to their program with PTSD. These programs often provide group therapy formats rather than individual therapy. This is done primarily to make the programs more cost effective and to make treatment available to more people who are suffering from PTSD. Unfortunately, this often means that the unique needs of each patient, especially those with complex PTSD and high levels of dissociative symptoms, are not adequately addressed by those programs. With respect to treating PTSD, my own clinical experience has shown that CBT is best suited for treating phobias and mild cases of PTSD that have low levels of dissociation.

DIALECTICAL BEHAVIOR THERAPY (DBT)

Dialectical Behavior Therapy [11] [12] is a modified form of CBT therapy that was developed by Marsha Linehan, specifically for the treatment of people who have *Borderline Personality Disorder* (BPD). However, since the majority of people with BPD have usually experienced significant amounts of trauma in their lives, many of them display symptoms of chronic, untreated PTSD. Thus, DBT could be considered to be a therapy for treating PTSD. The primary purpose of DBT is to reduce the high levels of self-defeating behavior, such as suicidal ideation, self-harm, impulsivity, and substance abuse that characterize people with borderline personalities. DBT helps people with BPD learn to recognize the emotional (dissociative) triggers of their behavior, to better regulate their emotions, and ultimately to reduce their self-defeating behavior and replace it with more adaptive ways of coping with stressful life situations.

An advantage of DBT is that Dr. Linehan has developed a standardized treatment manual for the therapy. The treatment has four essential components, Individual Therapy, Group Therapy, Team Consultation, and Phone Coaching. Because it is a team approach to therapy, it is a relatively labor and time intensive treatment that is best suited for mental health agencies with the necessary manpower to provide a DBT program. The major disadvantage of DBT is that it is often difficult to access agencies that offer a DBT program, primarily because of their cost, if you don't live in a larger population area. Also, because DBT is often a standardized program, it may not recognize the different levels of dissociative symptoms present in individuals with PTSD, and may not directly address their unique dissociative structure. Overall, DBT is best suited for treating Borderline Personality Disorder, the purpose for which it was originally intended.

EMOTION FOCUSED THERAPY (EFT)

Emotion Focused Therapy [13] [14] is a relatively short term form of therapy based on a recognition that human emotions play a necessary role in human survival. EFT proposes that our emotions act much like alarms, which provide essential feedback about how we are doing in our interactions with the world around us. The therapy has evolved from work by Les Greenberg and Sue Johnson beginning in the 1980's, and it is used for therapy with individuals, couples, and families. EFT differs dramatically from CBT, which is based on the premise that our thoughts drive our emotions and behavior, because EFT proposes exactly the opposite: that it is our emotions that drive our thoughts and actions. The goal of EFT therapy is to elicit, within the therapy session, the emotions that are attached to our current emotional conflicts. Once the emotions come to the surface, the task of therapy is to focus on the basic attachment needs that are being frustrated by the situation which is the focus of that session.

The major advantage of EFT is that it acknowledges that current emotional difficulties we are experiencing are related to our past emotional traumas. This is an essential assumption for any therapy for dissociation and PTSD. EFT is a highly focused therapy that is designed to be efficient. Research has shown that it can be effective for many people within 8 to 20 therapy sessions. The disadvantages of EFT are that it may not be as commonly available as CBT, because there may not be as many therapists in your area who have received the additional training to provide EFT. Another possible disadvantage is that additional psychodynamic therapy techniques (see below) may be required to treat cases of complex PTSD where dissociative symptoms are severe. With respect to treating PTSD, Emotion Focused Therapy (EFT) is likely most appropriate for treating cases of mild to moderate PTSD.

EYE MOVEMENT DESENSITIZATION AND REPROCESING (EMDR) THERAPY

Eye Movement Desensitization and Reprocessing Therapy, or EMDR,[15] [16] is also a relatively new therapy that was discovered accidentally by Francine Shapiro in the late 1980's. At the time, she discovered that her eyes began moving back and forth, out of her control, while she was experiencing some emotional trauma of her own. More importantly, she found that she could significantly reduce her anxiety if she purposely moved her eyes back and forth again. Based on that experience, she researched a new eye movement therapy and published the results in 1989. Because it was a dramatically new therapy that focused primarily on emotions, it was highly criticized within the established CBT community for many years, and is still criticized today by those who don't understand EMDR.

However, over the years, a volume of research has proven beyond a doubt that EMDR is an effective therapy for treating anxiety disorders, especially PTSD. In 2006, a study comparing the effectiveness of EMDR and CBT showed that both were equally effective in treating PTSD. [17] The authors noted that in the seven research studies that were compared, they could not determine if either EMDR or CBT was more effective for treating different groups of PTSD patients. Because people with mild PTSD and extremely complex PTSD were likely mixed together in the studies, it was not possible to determine if either CBT and EMDR was more appropriate for use in treating severe dissociation and complex PTSD.

However, given that the advocates of Cognitive Psychology and CBT generally do not acknowledge the existence of dissociation as a mental process, and therefore would not focus on treating your dissociation, this is a major problem if you're considering CBT for treating your complex PTSD symptoms. On the other hand, EMDR therapists are taught to recognize dissociation as being the most significant cluster of symptoms in PTSD, and they acknowledge that additional psychodynamic therapy is required, in combination with EMDR, to treat your dissociation and cases of complex PTSD.

The advantage of using EMDR for treating PTSD is that EMDR was developed specifically for treating PTSD, and it is a major breakthrough in treating the disorder. EMDR acknowledges and treats dissociation and the associated emotional and cognitive overload present in PTSD. It has a standardized treatment protocol, developed and fine-tuned over a twenty-five-year period, that all EMDR practitioners are required to adhere to. EMDR is a combination of Systematic Desensitization therapy and Cognitive Therapy, but therapy proceeds much more quickly by adding eye movements to stimulate both sides of your brain. Although EMDR initially used bilateral eye movements, it was discovered over the years that alternating sounds, or tapping from one side of the body to the other, can have the same effect as bilateral eye movements.

One of the major criticisms of EMDR in its early days was that it triggered dissociation and was, therefore, dangerous. However, as we have learned in this book, it is the nature of dissociation itself that can be potentially dangerous and difficult to treat. Because EMDR therapists are often dealing with the most complex and severe cases of PTSD, dissociation during therapy is much more likely to happen in those severe cases. Since EMDR therapists are more aware of dissociation, and they are better trained to deal with it when it occurs, this alleged disadvantage of EMDR is really one of its biggest assets.

One real disadvantage of EMDR is that extensive training is required to learn how to provide the therapy. It is rarely taught in graduate Psychology courses, which have long advocated CBT as the only effective evidence-based psychological treatment. Thus, you may find it more difficult to find an EMDR therapist in your area, particularly if you live in a smaller community. EMDR is also labor intensive. The length and cost of therapy increases dramatically as the severity of your dissociative symptoms increases. Furthermore, because additional psychodynamic therapy (see below) is usually combined with EMDR for treating complex PTSD cases, you will have a more difficult time finding an EMDR therapist with that kind of additional expertise and training. Overall, however, my years of clinical experience have taught me that EMDR is effective not only for treating phobias, but it is by far the most appropriate therapy for treating PTSD of all levels of severity.

PSYCHODYNAMIC THERAPY

Psychodynamic psychotherapy[18] developed in the latter years of the 19th century, beginning with the work of Sigmund Freud. The therapy quickly attracted the attention of many other early therapists such as Carl Jung, Alfred Adler, Otto Rank, and Melanie Klein. A more complete description of the history of Psychodynamic Therapy can be found in the Appendix of this book. However, to make a long story short, the therapy is based on the principle that we all have multiple unconscious mental processes, and that conflicts between those mental processes can cause people to experience emotional problems. Psychodynamic Therapy is the process of helping people to resolve those mental conflicts.

As mentioned in Chapter Four of this book, the concept of dissociation arose from psychodynamic theory. Therefore, it makes complete sense that Psychodynamic Therapy should be required to successfully treat the dissociative symptoms that you experience with your PTSD. The greater the degree of dissociation you experience, the greater the need for some kind of Psychodynamic Therapy to adequately treat PTSD.

The International Society for the Study of Trauma and Dissociation (ISSTD) published a set of Treatment Guidelines in 2011[19] for the treatment of Dissociative Identity Disorder (DID – sometimes known as Multiple Personality Disorder), which is characterized by severe Tertiary Dissociation. Although the guidelines specifically address DID, where the most serious symptoms of dissociation occur, they also provide a sound basis for treating complex PTSD, where high levels of severe Secondary Dissociation also occur.

The ISSTD guidelines recommend a phase-oriented approach to treating DID, very similar to what Pierre Janet, a pioneer in the study and treatment of dissociation and trauma, suggested almost a century ago.[20] The first, and possibly the most important phase of this approach to treating your PTSD, involves stabilizing and managing your symptoms. As mentioned above in the section on *Symptom Management*, we must ensure that you have the skills to manage your symptoms and keep yourself stable from day to day, before treatment of your dissociation and PTSD can begin. The second phase of treatment is where the various forms of psychological treatment mentioned above, including CBT or EMDR therapy, will help you to process and make sense of your traumatic memories. The third phase is where the dissociated mental processes discussed in Chapter Four are brought together with your growing understanding of your traumatic memories, so that your mental processes can resume working in a more integrated fashion. This third phase of treatment is known as *integration*. As this gradually occurs, the state of mental overload that caused your PTSD in the first place is gradually eliminated. The ISSTD guidelines strongly suggest that psychodynamic therapy is necessary to achieve this final phase of *integration*.

As you can see from the ISSTD treatment guidelines, you will need to find a therapist who can provide you with psychodynamic therapy, in addition to one or more of the other therapies mentioned above. EMDR and CBT therapies, which both have a long history of research evidence to show that they are effective in treating PTSD, are established therapies that can be used in combination with psychodynamic therapy to treat your PTSD symptoms.

WHERE CAN I GET TREATMENT?

Now that I've provided you with some different options for treating PTSD of varying degrees of severity, we are faced with the most critical part of treating the disorder: Where can I get the treatment I need?

I don't want to be discouraging or negative at this point, but I do need to be realistic. Finding and accessing quality treatment for your PTSD could be difficult, and you may have to be both persistent and creative in finding adequate treatment for your unique situation. You must consider many things when looking for PTSD treatment, including the professional qualifications of the mental health therapist, their training, what caused your PTSD symptoms, the severity and chronicity of your symptoms, and whether you have access to various kinds of funding for your treatment.

WHO IS QUALIFIED TO TREAT PTSD?

There are many different types of mental health professionals who may be qualified and licensed to treat mental health disorders, including PTSD, in the country or city where you live. Psychiatrists, psychologists, social workers, behavior therapists, and various types of psychotherapists may all theoretically have the necessary professional qualifications to treat PTSD. However, regardless of their degrees or professional qualifications, they all must have considerable extra training before they can provide you with adequate treatment for PTSD, especially if your dissociative symptoms are severe. Don't get hung up on looking for somebody with the highest degree or the most diplomas. I know plenty of well-trained social workers who have far more training and experience for treating PTSD than many psychologists or psychiatrists. So, when looking for PTSD treatment, make sure you ask therapists about how much extra training and experience they have in treating dissociation and severe cases of PTSD.

HOW WILL I PAY FOR TREATMENT?

The single biggest issue in finding PTSD treatment is funding. If your dissociative symptoms are extensive and your PTSD severe, your treatment is going to take much longer and is going to be more expensive. If you are fortunate and have a good income and good health benefits, it will make it much easier for you to access quality treatment for you PTSD symptoms. If you can't afford to pay for the treatment on your own, you are going to have to find other ways to fund your treatment.

The type of event that triggered your PTSD breakdown is an important issue in finding treatment. For example, if you were injured in the workplace, you may be eligible for having your treatment funded through the Worker's Compensation program in the province or state where you live. If your PTSD was caused by a motor vehicle accident, you may be eligible for funding through your automobile insurance. In some provinces and states, if your trauma resulted from somebody committing a criminal act, you might be eligible to apply for funding through Criminal Compensation programs. You should check to see whether your state or province has such a program. If your PTSD was a result of events you experienced in the military or as a first-responder, you may also be eligible for treatment. Sadly, this has not always been the case. Governments are only beginning to acknowledge the terrible toll that PTSD takes on our military personnel and first responders. Don't expect the system to automatically accept your PTSD diagnosis. Do expect that you may have to battle and persevere to have both your PTSD diagnosis and your right to treatment acknowledged.

Another source of funding for your PTSD treatment could be your private health insurance plan, especially if you live in the USA. Alternatively, if you live in a country which has universal health care, you may or may not be eligible for various levels of mental health treatment, depending on the country, state, or province where you live. The biggest problem with seeking treatment through insurance or government health plans is that they may have limits on either the number of treatment sessions or the amount of funding that is available for your treatment. Where treatment is available, you may have to settle for "cookie cutter" treatment programs that are designed to treat as many people as possible at one time, due to budget limitations within those programs. Also, many health insurance plans may only pay for treatment by psychologists or psychiatrists who are legally allowed to provide mental health diagnoses. This may limit your access to other therapists who are very experienced at treating dissociation and PTSD, but are not legally allowed to provide diagnoses.

A WORD ABOUT TREATMENT PROGRAMS

Quality, individualized treatment of your PTSD symptoms could be time-consuming and expensive, especially if your symptoms are severe and are longstanding. Government and institutional programs are often more interested in showing how many people they have treated, or how quickly they have been seen, as ways of demonstrating the effectiveness of their programs. They are interested in showing voters or shareholders that they are delivering services in the most cost effective manner. They are usually less interested in showing whether their treatment programs are actually making significant improvements in people's mental health status. This reality could make it difficult for you to receive individualized treatment that is tailored to the severity of your dissociation and PTSD symptoms. However, even if government and institutional programs might not be able to adequately treat moderate or severe cases of dissociation and PTSD, almost all of them should be able to teach you valuable skills for keeping yourself stable and for managing your symptoms until you can find adequate treatment.

SUMMARY

In summary, finding proper, effective treatment for your PTSD symptoms can be a long and frustrating ordeal. However, I urge you and your loved ones to be persistent and patient in your search to find the right therapist and the right treatment for you.

At this point, I realize that you may be feeling a bit disillusioned by how difficult it might be to find the right type of treatment and the right therapist for you. So, to help you, I've decided to create an online database on my website, http://www.drdr.ca/demystifying-ptsd.html, of treatment centers and therapists recommended by fellow readers. The database will be an ongoing work in progress, so keep checking it on a regular basis to see if somebody in your area has a recommendation that might be just right for your situation.

There has been great improvement over the past twenty-five or thirty years in the therapies that are available for treating PTSD, especially with the development of EMDR therapy and with ongoing improvement in our understanding and treatment of dissociation. Thus, there is hope. There is a very good chance that you can become symptom free if you remain patient, and if you manage to connect with a therapist near you who is properly trained and skilled at treating PTSD.

Appendix: A Brief History of Dissociation

In his 1988 book, *A Brief History of Time*, physicist Stephen Hawking took on the daunting task of explaining billions of years of the history of the universe in one book. Even more amazing, he managed to make it understandable for people like you and me. In comparison, my task of giving you a brief history of the roughly 125-year history of psychology is far less challenging. But for those of you who have read the first five chapters of this book, and who are still interested in why it took so long for psychologists to realize the importance of dissociation, I thought I'd give it a try.

Up to this point in our efforts to understand PTSD, I've told you that the most important factor in determining the severity of PTSD is dissociation. So logically, before we can help people like you to fully understand PTSD, we must help you to understand what we mean when we talk about dissociation, and where the concept originated.

THE NATURE OF DISSOCIATION

The biggest problem in explaining dissociation to people, as I did in Chapter Four of this book, is that, even though psychiatrists and some psychologists have talked about it for over a century, there has been very little systematic research on the subject over that period of time. In order to fully understand why there has been so little research on dissociation, especially since it is so important to our understanding of PTSD, it is necessary to understand a little bit about the history of both psychiatry and psychology over the past century.

SIGMUND FREUD AND PSYCHOANALYSIS

Love him or hate him and his theories, Sigmund Freud was the father of modern psychiatry and psychology. Freud was a medical doctor who was practicing in Vienna, Austria during the latter part of the Victorian era at the end of the 19th century. In his practice, he started noticing a disturbing trend in many of his patients, especially women. He noticed that a significant portion of his female patients were reporting a variety of physical ailments that were often vague and hard to diagnose. But he also noticed that many of those women were also extremely anxious and depressed, a condition that he called *neurosis.* Perhaps the most disturbing thing for Freud was that many of those patients began talking about sexual issues, something that was quite taboo in the very prim and proper days of Victorian Europe.

In order to make sense of this combination of physical ailments, neurosis, and sexual issues, Freud proposed a number of revolutionary theories[21] ranging from Psychosexual Fixations and Penis Envy, to Oedipal Love between mothers and sons. Even though most of his theories are largely rejected today, the most important part of his theories is that he proposed a direct link between active, dynamic mental processes and physical ailments. As a result, his theories were called *Psychodynamic Theories*, and the new science of Psychodynamic Psychiatry emerged. Between the end of the 19th century and the beginning of the First World War, many famous psychodynamic psychiatrists emerged who supported Freud's theories, while others such as Carl Jung and Pierre Janet proposed theories of their own.

The new wave of psychiatrists did their research by studying each one of their individual patients, and then trying to look for similarities and patterns in those patients. Once they saw patterns of symptoms and behavior, they formulated theories and new concepts to describe them. One of the first psychiatrists to focus specifically on dissociation was the French psychiatrist, Pierre Janet (1859-1947). Although he wasn't the first to use the word dissociation, he was the first to truly notice its importance while he was studying hypnosis and other states of altered consciousness. In 1886, Janet wrote about his observation that one of his patients appeared to show two distinctly different states of consciousness. Janet's doctoral dissertation in 1889 was the first major study of the phenomenon.

To make a long story very short, Janet proposed the existence of a number of automatic mental processes that can function outside of our awareness.[5] He also proposed that all of these unconscious mental processes must work together properly in an integrated fashion in order for each us to be psychologically healthy. Janet proposed that events in our lives can sometimes disturb the ability of our mental processes to work together, causing them to split apart. When that occurs, the different mental processes may struggle for control and will often interfere with each other, a phenomenon that Janet called dissociation.

Despite the great theoretical advances made by the psychoanalytic movement in treating mental health disorders, and despite Pierre Janet's enormous contribution to the world's understanding of dissociation, there was one serious limitation to their theories about unconscious mental processes: How do we test those theories in a systematic, scientific manner?

EXPERIMENTAL PSYCHOLOGY AND BEHAVIORISM

At about the same time that the psychoanalysts were formulating their theories from medical patients with mental health problems, another very different movement, known as Experimental Psychology, was taking hold in universities, first in Europe and then in North America. Experimental psychology uses the scientific method of creating experiments in order to discover factors that change behavior. A classic example of experimental psychology is the work of Ivan Pavlov,[22] whose experiments on Classical Conditioning led to discoveries that are still used today for helping people get over their anxiety and phobias, and whose research helped earn him a Nobel Prize in 1904.

Once psychologists began discovering factors in our environment that could change our behavior, they began creating therapies as early as 1911 to help people change their behaviors. The early Behaviorist Movement[3] was only interested in factors that existed in our environment or within our bodies that could influence our behavior. They were not concerned with the effect of human thought (cognitions) or emotions on our behavior. Behaviorism in psychology flourished through the 1940's and 1950's. During the 1950's, Joseph Wolpe, a South African psychiatrist, based his very successful *Systematic Desensitization*[8] therapy on the behavioral principles of counterconditioning developed earlier in the century by Pavlov. Systematic Desensitization is still used to this day for treating all kinds of phobias, and is probably the most used and most dependable treatment in all of psychology.

THE RISE OF COGNITIVE BEHAVIORAL THERAPY

By the late 1950's and 1960's, other psychologists such as Albert Ellis and Aaron Beck were becoming more concerned with the influence of human thinking on our behavior. Cognitive Psychologists[4] still relied almost exclusively on the scientific method to study human behavior. Unlike the behaviorists, they firmly believed that human thought was the driving force behind our emotions and our actions, so they developed therapies designed to change our thinking as a way of changing our moods, reducing anxiety, or changing the way we act. Their therapies became known as *Cognitive Behavioral Therapy*, [10] or CBT as it is often called today. It was a significant advance in the development of psychology because it recognized the important influence of our thoughts on our behavior, and it stimulated enormous amounts of psychological research.

At this point, you are probably asking yourself: What does the rise of CBT have to do with our discussion of dissociation and PTSD? I don't blame you for asking, because it's an extremely important question. The answer to your question lies in the Cognitive Psychologist's steadfast reliance on using the scientific method for doing their research. Human behavior and thoughts are easy to measure in scientific experiments, because it's easy for us to count specific types of behavior, and it's easy to ask people what they are thinking. But when it comes to emotions, things start to get murky.

Scientists can easily measure the end response of emotions on our moods and anxiety by interviewing people or having them fill out questionnaires. But it's extremely difficult to measure the dynamic mental processes in our brain that cause us to react emotionally. This created a huge problem for Cognitive Psychology researchers. So the easiest way to solve their problem was for them to simply declare that our emotions aren't important in driving our actions. They concluded that if mental processes such as dissociation can't be measured using the scientific method, they must not really exist. As a result, any further research on dissociation from the 1950's to the end of the century was highly discouraged in most schools of psychology, and CBT was proclaimed to be the *only* form of psychological therapy that was effective.

Dialectical Behavior Therapy (DBT) is a later development in the field of CBT that was developed by Marsha Linehan, specifically for treating people who have a very challenging condition known as Borderline Personality Disorder.[11][23] DBT has four essential components, Individual Therapy, Group Therapy, Team Consultation, and Phone Coaching. An advantage of DBT over traditional forms of CBT is that it is a team approach to therapy that is well suited to mental health agencies with the necessary manpower to provide a comprehensive DBT treatment program. However, like traditional CBT, DBT doesn't recognize dissociation as a significant mental process that must be addressed in the treatment of PTSD.

EMOTION FOCUSED THERAPY (EFT)

As I mentioned in Chapter 5, *Emotion Focused Therapy*[13] [14] is a relatively short term form of therapy based on a recognition that human emotions play a necessary role in human survival. It was developed, beginning in the 1980's by Les Greenberg and his colleague Sue Johnson. EFT was a significant advance in the field of psychology because Greenberg and Johnson were amongst the first psychologists to recognize that our emotions often play a more important role than our thoughts in driving behavior. They proposed that emotions act much like alarms, which provide essential feedback about how we're doing in our interactions with the world around us. From their theories, Greenberg and Johnson developed their new form of psychological treatment, *Emotion Focused Therapy*, which is used for treating individuals, couples, and families. The major contribution of EFT theory is that it started a movement towards developing psychological treatments that are backed by psychological research, like CBT, but are more focused on treating the emotions underlying our distress. EFT acknowledges that our emotional responses to current life difficulties are related to our past emotional traumas. This is an essential assumption for any therapy intended to treat dissociation and PTSD.

EYE MOVEMENT DESENSITIZATION AND REPROCESSING (EMDR) THERAPY

In Chapter 5, I also introduced you to *Eye Movement Desensitization and Reprocessing Therapy*, or EMDR,[15] [16] a relatively new therapy that was discovered accidentally by Francine Shapiro in the late 1980's. At the time, she discovered that her eyes began moving back and forth, out of her control, while she was experiencing some emotional trauma. More importantly, she found that she could significantly reduce her anxiety if she purposely moved her eyes back and forth again. Based on that experience, she researched a new eye movement therapy and published the results in 1989. Because it was a dramatically new therapy that focused primarily on emotions, it was highly criticized within the established CBT community for many years, and even still today.

One of the most frequent criticisms of EMDR by advocates of CBT was that EMDR caused dissociation and was, therefore, dangerous. This is rather an ironic criticism, given that CBT purists generally don't like to acknowledge the existence of unconscious mental processes such as dissociation. There was, however, some validity to their criticism.

EMDR therapists quickly learned that the eye movements (bilateral brain stimulation) of EMDR were very good at activating the emotions attached to our traumatic memories. However, for people with histories of severe trauma and severe dissociation, the emotions could activate too quickly, and the emotional responses could be overwhelming for some patients. Rather than be deterred by this obstacle, EMDR therapists realized that the solution was not to abandon EMDR. Instead, advocates of EMDR realized they needed to revive the long-dormant research on dissociation. They reasoned that they needed to better understand the underlying unconscious mental processes involved in dissociation, in order to improve EMDR therapy.

RE-EMERGENCE OF PSYCHODYNAMIC RESEARCH AND THERAPY

In 1984, a number of doctors and psychologists in the United States formed the *International Society for the Study of Multiple Personalities and Dissociation.*[24] It was a non-profit association devoted to furthering research and scientific understanding of trauma-based disorders such as PTSD, Multiple Personality Disorder, (now known as *Dissociative Identity Disorder or DID*), and other Dissociative Disorders. Now known as the *International Society for the Study of Trauma and Dissociation* (ISSTD), the society publishes a peer-reviewed scientific journal, *The Journal of Trauma and Dissociation*. More importantly, the ISSTD has also published guidelines for treating DID, which have become the roadmap for treating people with severe PTSD and DID.[19]

It is no coincidence that the founding of the ISSTD occurred at about the same time that Greenberg and Johnson were developing the theories that led them to develop *Emotion Focused Therapy*. Long neglected during the years that psychology was dominated by the Behaviorists and by Cognitive Behavioral psychology, therapists who treated people with PTSD and other dissociative disorders were looking for better tools to treat people affected by these severe disorders. A key recommendation in the ISSTD Guidelines for treating DID and severe dissociative disorders, is the need to use some form of Psychodynamic Therapy. With that recommendation, psychology came full circle and re-established the importance of century-old dissociation as the primary problem in trauma-based disorders.

Today, modern researchers continue to work on expanding our knowledge of dissociation. For example, Van der Hart and colleagues[6] have developed a theory of *Structural Dissociation*. Their theory provides a defined structure for understanding dissociation, yet the structure is flexible enough to allow therapists to vary the unique nature of dissociation for every person affected by PTSD or other dissociative disorders. When combined with newer emotion-based therapies such as EMDR, therapists now have a powerful tool for managing and understanding a patient's dissociation, allowing EMDR to be safer and more effective than ever.

What's amazing about the *Structural Dissociation* model, is that clients with extensive dissociation quickly grasp the model because it fits so closely with their daily experience of dissociation. Once they learn to understand and trust the model, it allows them to proceed with EMDR or other therapies with more confidence, and it provides a more complete treatment of their PTSD.

SUMMARY

As you can see from our brief history of dissociation, the science of psychology has come full circle over the 125 years. Some amazing insights by the pioneers of psychology and psychiatry into trauma and dissociation, swept aside by the events of World War I and the domination of experimental psychology for most of the twentieth century, have re-emerged again in the twenty-first century. As psychologists began shifting their attention to the study of emotions, they re-introduced the world to the nature of dissociation. By doing so, they added to what we discovered from the Behaviorist and Cognitive Behavioral perspectives over the past century, enriching the science of psychology and greatly improving our ability to treat challenging disorders such as PTSD, DID, and other dissociative disorders. I'm not saying these disorders are suddenly easy to treat now – they definitely are not. But unlocking the century-long mystery surrounding dissociation has given us a key to help demystify devastating disorders such as PTSD and DID.

References

1. **American Psychiatric Association.** *Diagnostic and Statistical Manual of Mental Disorders.* 5th. Arlington : American Psychiatric Association Publishing, 2013.

2. **European Society for Traumatic Stress Studies.** ICD10 PTSD. *European Society for Traumatic Stress Studies.* [Online] 04 05, 2016. [Cited: 04 05, 2016.] https://www.estss.org/learn-about-trauma/icd10/.

3. **Wikipedia.** Behaviorism. *Wikipedia: The Free Encyclopedia.* [Online] March 22, 2016. [Cited: March 24, 2016.] https://en.wikipedia.org/wiki/Behaviorism.

4. **Wikipedia**. Cognitive Psychology. *Wikipedia: The Free Encyclopedia.* [Online] March 23, 2016. [Cited: March 24, 2016.]
 https://en.wikipedia.org/wiki/Cognitive_psychology.

5. *The Dissociation Theory of Pierre Janet.* **van der Hart, Onno and Horst, Rutger.** Springer, 1989, Journal of Traumatic Stress, Vol. 2, pp. 397-412.

6. **van der Hart, Onno, Nijenhuis, Ellert R.S. and Steele, Kathy.** *The Haunted Self: Structural Dissociation and the Treatment of Chronic Traumatization.* New York : W.W. Norton & Company, 2006.

7. **Petri, Daniel** [Director]. *Sybil.* [TV Mini-Series]. Schreiber, F.R. and Stern, S. 1976.

8. **Wikipedia.** Systematic Desensitization. *Wikipedia, The Free Encyclopedia.* [Online] 02 29, 2016. [Cited: 04 04, 2016.] https://en.wikipedia.org/wiki/Systematic_
desensitization.

9. **Wikipedia**. Cognitive Therapy. *Wikipedia, The Free Encyclopedia.* [Online] 03 27, 2016. [Cited: 04 05, 2016.] https://en.wikipedia.org/wiki/Cognitive_therapy.

10. **Wikipedia**. Cognitive Behavioral Therapy. *Wikipedia, The Free Encyclopedia.* [Online] 03 23, 2016. [Cited: 04 04, 2016.]https://en.wikipedia.org/wiki/Cognitive_behavioral_ therapy.

11. **Linehan, Marsha.** *Cognitive-Behavioral Treatment of Borderline Personality Disorder.* New York: The Guilford Press, 1993.

12. **Wikipedia.** Dialectical Behavior Therapy. *Wikipedia: The Free Encyclopedia.* [Online] February 28, 2016. [Cited: March 24,2016.]
https://en.wikipedia.org/wiki/
Dialectical_behavior_therapy.

13. **Greenberg, Leslie S. and Paivio, Sandra C.** *Working With Emotions in Psychotherapy.* New York: The Guilford Press, 1997.

14. **Wikipedia.** Emotionally Focused Therapy. *Wikipedia, The Free Encylopedia.* [Online] 03 01, 2016. [Cited: 04 04, 2016.] https://en.wikipedia.org/wiki/
Emotionally_focused_therapy.

15. **Shapiro, Francine and Forrest, Margot S.** *EMDR: The Breakthrough Therapy for Overcoming Anxiety, Stress, and Trauma.* New York: Basic Books, 1997.

16. **Wikipedia.** Eye Movement Desensitization and Reprocessing. *Wikipedia, The Free Encylcopedia.* [Online] 04 04, 2016. [Cited: 04 04, 2016.] https://en.wikipedia.org/wiki/Eye_movement_ desensitization_and_reprocessing.

17. *Comparing the Efficacy of EMDR and Trauma-Focused Cognitive-Behavioral Therapy in the Treatment of PTSD: A Meta-Analytic Study.* **Seidler, Guenter H. and Wagner, Frank E.** Cambridge, UK: Cambridge University Press, 11 2006, Psychological Medicine, Vol. 36, pp. 1515-1522.

18. **Wikipedia.** Psychodynamic Psychotherapy. *Wikipedia, The Free Encyclopedia.* [Online] 04 02, 2016. [Cited: 04 04, 2016.] https://en.wikipedia.org/wiki/Psychodynamic_ psychotherapy.

19. **International Society for the Study of Trauma and Dissociation.** Adult Treatment Guidelines. *International Society for the Study of Trauma and Dissociation.* [Online] 03 03, 2011. [Cited: 04 12, 2016.] http://www.isst-d.org/default.asp?contentID=49.

20. *Pierre Janet's Treatment of Post-traumatic Stress.* **van der hart, Onno, Brown, Paul, and van der Kolk, Bessel A.** International Society for Traumatic Stress Studies, 10 1989, Journal of Traumatic Stress, Vol. 2, pp. 379-395.

21. **Wikipedia.** Sigmund Freud. *Wikipedia, the Free Encyclopedia.* [Online] July 1, 2016. [Cited: July 1, 2016.] https://en.wikipedia.org/wiki/Sigmund_Freud.

22. **Wikipedia**. Ivan Pavlov. *Wikipedia, The Free Encyclopedia.* [Online] 03 11, 2016. [Cited: 03 11, 2016.] https://en.wikipedia.org/wiki/Ivan_Pavlov.

23. **Linehan, Marsha M.** *DBT Skills Training Manual, Second Edition.* New York: The Guilford Press, 2015.

24. **Wikipedia.** International Society for the Study of Trauma and Dissociation. *Wikipedia, the Free Encyclopedia.* [Online] 04 14, 2016. [Cited: 04 21, 2016.] https://en.wikipedia.org/wiki/International_Society_for_
the_Study_of_Trauma_and_Dissociation.

25. **Bremner, Douglas J. M.D.** The Invisible Epidemic: Post-Traumatic Stress Disorder, Memory and the Brain. *The Doctor Will See You Now.* [Online] 08 01, 2011. [Cited: 04 28, 2012.]
http://www.thedoctorwillseeyounow.com/content/
stress/art1964.html.

26. **Mental Health America.** Dissociation and Dissociative Disorders. *Mental Health America.* [Online] 04 05, 2016. [Cited: 04 05, 2016.]
http://www.mentalhealthamerica.net/conditions/
dissociation-and-dissociative-disorders.

EMDR Resources

U.S.A.

EMDR International Association (EMDRIA)
5806 Mesa Drive, Suite 360
Austin, TX 78731
Tel +1 (866) 451-5200
Fax +1 (512) 451-5256
Email: info@emdria.org
Website: http://www.emdria.org/

CANADA

EMDR Canada
P.O. Box 711, Succ. Lachute,
Lachute (QC) J8H 4G4 Canada
Tel: +1 (450) 537-1554
Fax number: +1 (450) 537-1441
Website: https://emdrcanada.org/

EUROPE

EMDR Europe
Website: http://www.emdr-europe.org/

AUSTRALIA

EMDR Australia (EMDRAA)
Website: http://emdraa.org/

NEW ZEALAND

Website: http://www.emdr.org.nz/

PTSD Treatment Resources

Visit Dr. Jones' website below for a dynamic, interactive database of treatment centers and therapists suggested by other readers. Dr. Jones and ANP Publishing make no claims or representations about the qualifications or effectiveness of any of these treatment centers or therapists, so keep in mind that the onus is on you to check out these recommendations on your own, to determine if the treatment center or therapist is appropriate for your unique situation and PTSD symptoms.

http://www.drdr.ca/demystifying-ptsd.html